Green Organic Kitchen cleaners Guide For Mothers: Your Step BY Step DIY Guide On Making Organic Cleaning Disinfectant, That Kills Bacteria, Viruses, Fungi, And Other Germs Quickly in Less Than 5 Minutes; Using The "SCEM + CBC" System.

Jane Mark

CONTENTS

Everybody is now more particular about their health, especially since the outbreak of this deadly pandemic called COVID 19.

Attention on the product used in our home is not always put into consideration. Many products use in the cleaning of our home are usually toxic to our health and environment without the user knowing.

From the way we grew up, product marketers got our attention that the product we can use to clean our home must be those expensive ones. All of these are false.

Read this; you can clean your home with a product done by yourself with little dollars in your hand.

Not only is making this non-toxic product cheaper, but it is also easy to make. So, please forget the irony product marketers have downloaded you with and begin to change your mindset on the possibilities that are existing in preparing organic cleaning agents.

Our desire as moms is to make our home clean using a cleaning agent. However, consideration is placed on maintaining a healthy environment.

I don't know about; I always want to live my environment healthy, better than the way I found it. From my experiences as a mom, I discovered that most of the products I got from the market were not hygienic to the environment, which left me with no option than to look for a better solution.

I started to produce my own natural homemade cleaning agent that serves as a remedy to my problem.

Surprisingly, those products I did for my personal use were from organic raw materials that are cheap, non-toxic, and very effective in cleaning the house. Now the key factor there was me trying to combine each of the raw materials at a required amount to produce the result I need.

I believe if you are a lover of a natural lifestyle, you will get the gist I am passing across to you. I know you didn't make that choice of living a natural lifestyle overnight. Living a life full of vigour is all filled with responsibility which you have to take personally.

The organic cleaning recipes in this book is based on your regular cleaning approaches. But, if you feel it is not enough for you, you will have to adjust the ideas in this book to feet your choice.

But before, you go into the recipe in this book; I will like you to go through the next chapter has I explain the cleaning industry.

I so much believe you will learn alot as you go through this easy to make home cleaning agents that are non-toxic and efficient.

One of the significant factors about natural cleaning products is the fact you don't have to use a customized package for it. You can use any bottle of your choice to package it, which is unlike the commercial cleaning agent that is toxic.

If staying fit doesn't come with a significant cost from our pocket, then the same can be for our health and environment.

You don't need many things to get your home clean, but what you need is soap, water in addition to the basic recipe I will be listing in this book.
So, keep going to see the mind-blowing recipes you can use to clean your home. Don't forget that there is an option for you so if you are just starting, all you have to do is to choose the simple recipe, and with the time you make use of the recipe that is more advance.

From the idea in this book, you can try other concoction with the idea in this book.

Commercial cleaning agent companies has made us believe every product that makes it into the market has passed the test of standard and we can now use it for anything we want to do without it harming us

You want to buy a product, you check the label and what you see is misleading because it has made us believe what is written in the product is safe for use.

Some of the issues I have against this company are;

1. These companies are usually restricted to list all the ingredients used in making their cleaning product. Thus, they only list the primary ingredient use for their production.

Read this, the American Cleaning Institute, the Consumer Specialty Products Association, and the Canadian Consumer Specialty Products Association establish a program in 2010 whose aim is to protect the every manufacturing interest in respect to their product manufacturing process, packaging, distribution, and sale to various consumers, which are households.

For those that decide to list this ingredient, not all the ingredient are included in the list.

Some of this ingredient are toxic and they might decide to include just one, the rest are classified as trade secrets according to Lorie Dwornick, who is an educational researcher, and activist, 2002

In 2010, the International Fragrance Association said that companies are on their own will to disclose the formula for their product or not.

Therefore, this keeps you with no option than to use what you don't know if it is safe or not.

2. Some of this product when used overtime result to an accumulated toxin in the body, which result in secondary health issue in our body.

For you to overcome this health challenge that might not occur immediately, you have to take it as a responsibility to act upon this information in this book.

Don't wait for later, investigate every product you get in this market because they have the possibility of causing health issues when used for a long period.

Take for instance, whoever thought that mercury which people were using in the workplace can ever result in mercury poisoning until it happened.

3. Some of this chemical can be a pro-carcinogenic substance, which when inhaled or absorbed by the skin during usage can result in cancer.

What I mean by pro-carcinogenic is, this cleaning agent on their or on or two of its ingredients can stimulate cancer formation activity of the body, thereby making one more prone to cancer.

Therefore, while using this commercial cleaning agent, take note that cancer still exists.

4. One of the systems in our body that is very vital in proper day to day activities is the endocrine system. Some of these commercial products can interrupt the endocrine function of the body.
What this endocrine interrupter does is they mal the function of the endocrine system, resulting in one health challenge or the other. According to the 2005 guide to cancer and its treatment by Thomson and Jacqueline such health challenge include cancer, birth defect, and deformation of organs controlled by the endocrine system.

5. Some of these substances can be detrimental to the body's central nervous system. Affecting the neurons of the body. Thus, this chemical can be referred to as neurotoxins. According to a TerraChoice study from 2009 to 2010, an example of deformities encountered as a result of the neurotoxins is epilepsy, dementia, which is among others.

6. Some of this product has cautionary labels on them, which the meaning of these labels is not well defined. Thus making it dangerous for the consumers to understand.

By this, you are put on a risk of using more than required, which can be harmful to your health.

Have you Had of GreenWashing?

Presumably, you must have heard about greenwashing or not.

But which every day, I will tell you what greenwashing is.

The word got its origin to explain practices of the hotel industry in 1986. Hotels usually practice the act of placing placards in front of their bathroom. The essence of this was to promote the conservation of water by encouraging their visitor or customers to use towels.

When you look at it critically, you will discover that it is mainly there to increase the fund of the hotel rather than to preserve the environment as suppose.

During the period, the products bought are expensive, sometimes ineffective, by this many of the company wants the consumer to think that natural products are not effective in cleaning so that attention will be shifted in getting manufactured cleaners.

How do these companies achieve their aim?

1. Most of this company didn't add toxic chemical use in the production of their product. Even though the Consumer Product Safety Commission (CPSC) advocates that a commercial company should add or list the key ingredients used in making their product. So, this company will list those chemicals labeled non-toxic in the ingredient list of Consumer Product Safety Commission (CPSC) and make their product non-toxic product.

2. They're no standard rule that specifies the use of a natural ingredient in the production of non-consumable items by the United States Department of Agriculture (USDA). Unlike the specification given for consumable products like meat and poultry.

So, Manufacturing companies might decide to label their ingredient natural to their discretion.

3. Since there is no standard out there that can define the environmentally friendliness of a product, therefore environmental friendliness of any of these commercial products cannot be certified.
4. for you to say a product is biodegradable. When exposing to moisture, air, micro-organism like bacteria, air it must degrade to a non-harmful substance in a short period, according to the Federal Trade Commission (FTC) guidelines.

But keen attention is not paid to this, as a company on their discretion can say their product is biodegradable or not.

Another agency that ensures the product is certified biodegradable is SCS, which they arrive through standard research methodology and provision of information by the company.

But, what so many companies do is this, they make use of misleading labels to greenwash their product.

In 2010, 5, 296 products were evaluated for biodegradability, out of all, 265 products were biodegradably certified according to the TerraChioce survey. So, the question now is, what happens to the remaining ones that were not certified but have always been in the market.

The answer is, they are greenwash products.

How Cleaning Product is green Wash by Companies

The questions are which company doesn't want to go green?

Of course known, since they are making lots of money at the detriment to the earth of their customers and the safety of the environment.

Certifying a company as a company producing the eco-friendly product is such a big achievement that the company has it means the company is well accredited for the proper product, which means more sales and profit.

In 2004 Glaser reported that an independent researcher at Environmental Working Group (EWG) did a review on 2000 + cleaning products. They discovered that those product acclaimed to be non-toxic contain in them chemical ingredient that is toxic to the body and environment.

How Cleaning product is Greenwashed

So I will be given you some clue on how cleaning products are greenwashed by the manufacturer.

They are as follows as collected from the EWG Cleaners Database Hall of Shame;

When you see a labeled purpose cleaner product is in a spray bottle. They are packaged as non-toxic and biodegradable.

The nozzle of the spray indicates that you will use it without diluting it since it is in the form of a spray. But, if you should check the company website, they usually recommend you dilute it, but because of the package it came with, it becomes difficult for you to follow.

Using it without diluting can be detrimental to your health.

But, It is the same product that is label as a non-toxic cleaner. But, in the later run, it contains an ingredient that affects the red blood cell and that is irritant to the skin.

Some of the products sold in package aerosol form are usually can be breathed into the body easily or the skin can absorb it. An example of It is cleaner use to clean the oven. Some of this product contains some amount of potassium hydroxide or sodium, which can burn the lungs, eyes, and skin.

Disinfectant in the form of a powder used as a cleaner contains as high as 144+ chemicals, which some of these chemicals can cause asthma, reproductive anomalies, and cancer.

Some of these chemicals are not listed in the label. Such chemical are formaldehyde, toluene, chloroform, and benzene

Just like we have explained before, many companies don't list all the ingredients they use for their product.

Meanwhile on norm manufacturers are told to prove that their product is non-toxic. However, there is usually an oversight of the ingredient used in the production of this product. Most times the chemicals are not controlled by agencies.

A Part to Play

It is your responsibility to make sure the cleaner product you are using is the right kind of product that would not cause harm to you.

That is why I am advocating for you to make use of a homemade cleaning agent that is non-toxic to the body.

So to be on a safer side, scrutinize the product you buy, either using your money or getting someone to do it for you.

Using your money implies getting from a company that lists all the ingredients use in making their product or you make your product by yourself.

You can also apply the principle of contacting the company yourself, telling them to give you the list of the ingredient they use to produce their product.

You can start on your own by telling people in your office, school, or area you stay to start using homemade cleaning products using non-toxic ingredients.

1. People think that nature made cleaning agents are not as active as the cleaning agent made using chemical agents that are not natural.

This idea is what commercial companies have put on you people in a bit to make more money for themselves.

2. The product produce by manufacturing companies has passed through a well-approved test and that of the naturally produced ones have not.

Due to the lapses by law enforcement agencies to follow this law, they made us believe that It is true.

3. They made us believe that the smell of the commercially made product is proportionate to how effective the product it.

However, you should know that cleaners normally should not have a smell, if at all it does it is because of this presence of fragrance in the products

4. Natural Homemade clean can't clean as effectively as the one produced by companies out there.

Well, It is force, the ability of your homemade cleaner to clean effectively depends on the recipe you combine to give you what you want.

5. Natural Homemade product does not hat the ability to kill germs.

But the case is different here, in fact, it has is shown that using vinegar and hydrogen peroxide effective in cleaning bacteria and viruses even more effective than the cleaner manufactured from the lab.

6. Natural Homemade clean off course which is non-toxic are higher in terms of cost as opposed to those manufactured by companies.

Meanwhile, It is a lie, right in your house, you can produce your cleaning product in your house without stress.

7. While cleaning it takes me more time and energy to finish cleaning when using a homemade natural product. I will tell you that is false.

Just use the right combination of natural products and before you know it within a minute you are done with your cleaning.

8. The recipe to make a homemade natural product is usually difficult to get thus making its production difficult.

Well, that is also a lie; the product ingredient is available everywhere. You can get it without stress.

9. It is no difference between the chemical used in making a natural homemade cleaner and that use by the manufacturing company.

That is one of the myths they have made us believe.

Well, it will also let you know that it is false.

The first principle is you starting with the cleaning.

I know it is not easy changing your cleaning product from the ones you buy in the market to the ones you do yourself naturally from home.

But, mind you, It is one of the best decisions you can make as a wife, spinster, bachelor, or otherwise.

As your health is of utmost importance to anything else.

Don't be concerned with where to get the ingredient you will use for your cleaning. As we proceed, you will come to discover that most of this ingredient is right there in your kitchen.

However, if they are not there, you can still find them quickly at every local grocery store in your vicinity.

So, the goal of this book is to help you save money and teach you how to make homemade natural, non-toxic cleaning products.

Chemistry Involve

To produce a cleaner product, you have to understand the chemistry involved in its production.

Even manufacturing company that is the process they make use of when doing their production.

One of the critical factors we have to look at is the primary and acidic property of the product.

So, the question is, is the product or ingredient used to produce the product acidic or alkaline?

So, what our cleaning agent does is to bring the stained surface to a pH of 7.

Like when you look at some of the cleaning agents, you will notice that chemical like vinegar and lemon are naturally acidic. At the same time, substances like baking soda is an essential natural substance.

White acidic vinegar can neutralize stains and reduce the effect of the mineral in the stains. However, we still have apple cider vinegar, which I will not recommend for you to use to add more stain to the already existing one.

Alkaline natural cleaning homemade agent can neutralize stain; however, the mineral part of its constituent can cause abrasion. But, notwithstanding, when mix in the right proportion will perform magic in cleaning stains.

As we progress, you will come to understand better.

The second principle is you understanding the necessary supplies you will need for you to make your green kitchen cleaner.

Part of what we will be exploring is some standard cleaning suppliers, and I know you will find this very interesting. Even though some you already know, while some you don't.

Each day so many cleaning products are washed into the drain. Part of this remains in the drainage because of the toxic substance in the product.

The question now is, what happens to these substances when they are washed into the rivers?

Of course, they go through the food chain, which eventually harms us on the latter on.

However, It is not our focus now; what we will be considering is this: the ingredient we are going to be using to make our homemade cleaners are easy to get and use. But don't allow the list of ingredients stop you from continuing your practice as It is your first test.

So, I advise you to begin with the ones you already have in your house, and as you continue, you can begin trying more recipes for yourself.

Some of the ingredients you may probably have now are;

1. White vinegar

2. Baking soda

3. Castile soap

What you will help me do right now is to put those ingredients into a tea tree oil to make a potent cleaning powder.

Baking Soda

Other names: bicarbonate of soda.

Chemistry: an alkaline base that reacts with acids.

Where to get it: Grocery store.

Natural Occurrence: They can be found even in the human body, where they form a significant component of bile.

White Distilled Vinegar

Chemistry: an alkaline base that reacts with acids.

Where to get it: Grocery store.

Lemon Juice

Chemistry: It is acidic.

Where to get it: Grocery store.

Function: it can help to clean grease, aid the shining of the surface, and kills mould.

Soap vs Detergent

Chemistry: Detergent is made from petroleum distillates while the soap is made from saponin, using natural oil like olive oil.

Where to get it: Grocery store.

Uses: both detergent and soap are good at cleaning grease. However, detergent is dangerous as some of its ingredients are non-biodegradable, thus harming wildlife and man.

Borax

Other names: sodium tetraborate decahydrate, disodium tetraborate, or Sodium borate.

Chemistry: an alkaline base that reacts with acids.

Where to get it: Grocery store.

Note that you have to take when using borax to avoid inhaling the fine particles of the substance to avoid respiratory irritation

Hydrogen Peroxide

Other names: bicarbonate of soda.

Chemistry: an alkaline base that reacts with acids.

Where to get it: Grocery store.

Natural Occurrence: They can be found even in the human body, where they form a significant component of bile.

Hydrogen peroxide (H_2O_2) is a strong oxidizer, making it useful for bleaching and cleaning aid. It occurs naturally in low concentrations in nature as a by-product of oxidative metabolism in living organisms. Hydrogen peroxide is considered a highly reactive oxygen species. Concentrated hydrogen peroxide solutions are sometimes used as a rocket propellant. Diluted 3 per cent solutions are sold to the public and used for cleaning. Look for hydrogen peroxide in the personal care section of your grocery store.

Vodka

Where to get it: you can get it anywhere, alcohol is sold.

That can be a perfect ingredient for making extracts or in sprays where the carrier medium is used to make it quickly evaporate.

Washing Soda

Other names: It is also called soda ash or soda crystals or sodium carbonate.

Uses: it is used to soften water domestically, preventing magnesium and calcium ions in hard water to bond with detergent.

It can be used to remove stains like grease oil that are difficult to remove.

Water

One of the primary ingredients for the cleaning recipe is water. It is easily seen everywhere. But you should know that not all forms of water are useful. Some are filtered, which is better in cleaning appliances, but if it is hard, it won't be an excellent choice to use it. So the best thing for you to do is to look for the best for you to use.

Witch Hazel

Witch Hazel is an extract from the shrub of *Hamamelis virginiana.* It is sold as a product in a grocery store.

The third secret in my formula is the choice of essential oil I am using.

Essential Oils are natural plant extracts gotten from shrubs, herbs, trees, grasses, and flowers through various chemical processes like solvent extraction, distillation, evaporation, or even expression.

This product is safer to use because it will not accumulate in our body, unlike the artificial cleaning agents that are dangerous to our bodies.

The beauty of this oil is they have some biological property that fights against micro-organisms like fungi, bacteria, and viruses. However, this depends on the type of essential oil.

This should not permit you to misuse this oil as some of them are concentrated, thus becoming harmful to your skin; thus this call for you to dilute it with a carrier oil that will serve as a base.

As we continue in this book, we shall be looking at this various essential oil you can use.

You can do your research for others too, as they are thousands of them available.

Makes sure these oils are kept out of reach of children. To get already prepared essential oil that is made from a natural product, you can check 100% Natural Multi-purpose Cleaner

Let us now go into the essential oil we are talking about:

Grapefruit Oil

It is known as *Citrus paradise.*

It has a pleasant citrus scent.

It can combine very well with other essential oil.

It is used as an antiseptic and anti-bacterial agent.

If you want to add good scents to your essential oil, you should consider using lemon oil, for a floral scent, use ylang ylang oil, and for woodsy scent, use pine oil.

Sunflower Oil

It is called *Helianthus annuus*. Its colour is light amber. It is used in several ways apart from cleaning, which is a homemade recipe. You can get it in a grocery store.

Olive Oil

It is also called *Olea europaea.* You can see it everywhere; It is because of its culinary applications, majorly with Mediterranean recipes. You can use it as a homemade cleaning agent. You can get it in a grocery store.

Bergamot oil

It is also called *Citrus bergamia*. It is cold-pressed from bergamot orange fruit rind. It can be used as a fragrance, as seen in the fragrance industry. Apart from its cleaning ability, it is an *Analgesic, anti-bacterial, antiseptic, antispasmodic* agent.

Ylang Ylang Oil

It is also called *Cananga odorata*. It has a beautiful floral scent; it is combined with any essential oil. It is the right agent that can be used to fight bacteria, fungi, and inflammation.

Catnip Oil

Its other name is *Nepeta cataria*. It is used as a natural insect repellant. It's known for its ability to excite cats, thus can act as a sedative. It can be used to treat insect bites. Since it is related to mint, it has a mint-like aroma.

Chamomile Oil, German

It is also known as *Matricaria recutita*. Serve as a significant ingredient in body care products.

It is a perfect cleaning agent and also an anti-bacterial and antifungal agent.

You can use it in combination with other essential oil. Other properties include Analgesic, anti-bacterial, antifungal, anti-inflammatory, and antispasmodic.

Cedar Oil

It is also called *Juniperus virginiana.*
It can repel insects.
It is the right body care product.
It has a woodsy scent that blends with other wood-derived essential oils.
You can use it to clean and disinfect your home. It is an excellent antimicrobial, anti-bacterial, antifungal agent.

Cinnamon Bark Oil

It is also called *Cinnamomum zeylanicum.* It is an excellent natural essential oil for disinfecting surfaces because of its Analgesic, anti-bacterial, antifungal, anti-inflammatory, antimicrobial, antispasmodic, disinfectant.

Chamomile Oil, Roman

It is also called *Anthemis nobilis.*

Roman chamomile has a sweet scent with a hint of apples.

It is used in many natural body care products and also works well in aromatherapy. Blends with Roman chamomile are an excellent choice for air diffusion— Analgesic, anti-bacterial, anti-inflammatory, antimicrobial, antiseptic, antispasmodic.

Citronella Oil

It is also called *Cymbopogon winterianus.* It is a natural insect repellant that is used as a home remedy. It is used in combination with other essential oil.

Jasmine Absolute Oil

It is also called *Jasminum grandiflorum.*

The oil has an unforgettable story in the fragrance industry. It is combined with other essential oil. It has anti-inflammatory and Analgesic.

Lavender Oil

It is also called *Lavendula angustifolia.* It is one of the famous oil use as household oil. It is used as an antiseptic and for relieving pain from minor stings and bites. It is a good relaxer, that is what it is known for. Other properties are antispasmodic, antifungal, anti-inflammatory, and antimicrobial.

Lemon Eucalyptus Oil

It is also called *Eucalyptus citriodora.*
It is also used in the fragrance industry.
It has been discovered that it is a good popular bug repellant.
It has a light lemon scent, and this blends well with other oil.

Juniper Oil

Its other name is *Juniperus communis.* This oil is used to purify the air, and it is also be used as insect repellents.

It has analgesic, antiseptic, antimicrobial, and antispasmodic properties.

Lemon Oil

It is also called *Citrus limon*.
It has good cleaning ability.
It is a regular home cleaning addition because of its scent. It has analgesic, antiseptic, antimicrobial, and antispasmodic properties.

Lemon Balm Oil

It is also known as *Melissa officinalis*. It has a calming effect, and it is an insect repellant. It is popularly used in natural medicine. It has cleaning properties. Thus it can be added to any natural cleaning agent to enhance their effectiveness. It has analgesic, antiseptic, antimicrobial, and antispasmodic properties.

Lemongrass Oil

It is also called *cymbopogon flexuosus*. It is popularly known for its insect repellant property. Lemongrass essential oil has received recent exposure for its use as a natural insect repellent. Its property made it possible to be an additional cleaning agent.

.

Lime Oil

It is also called *Citrus aurantifolia*. It has a similar function that has lemon oil.

Oregano Oil

It is also known as *Origanum vulgare*. This essential oil works very well in fighting against micro-organisms like parasites, fungi, and bacteria. This oil blend very well with wood-based essential oil.

Orange (Sweet) Oil

It is also known as *Citrus sinensis*. This essential oil contains 90 % of limonene, one of the significant ingredients in homemade cleaners. It has analgesic, antiseptic, antimicrobial, and antispasmodic properties.

Sage Oil

It is also known as *Salvia officinalis*. It is popular because of its healing property; thus, the name *Salvia* meaning "health." However, pregnant and lactating women should take care when taking this essential oil. It has analgesic, antiseptic, antimicrobial, and antispasmodic properties.

Tea Tree Oil

It is also known as *Melaleuca alternifolia*. You can easily find this in the home of everyone cleaning their home with natural oil. It is because of its natural cleaning ability. It is an all-purpose essential oil and, when diluted, can work perfectly well. It has analgesic, antiseptic, antimicrobial, and antispasmodic properties. There is a famous story that Australian soldiers are given a tea tree to help them fight against infections.

Thyme Oil

It is also called *Thymus vulgaris*.
It is well known for its disinfectant and antiseptic properties.
You can use it in combination with other essential oil.

Clove Bud Oil

It is also known as *Syzygium aromaticum*. It is a perfect natural medicine that helps fight against viruses and diseases. Thus, it will be useful to combine it with other cleaning agents to produce the maximum result.

Eucalyptus Oil

It is also known as *Eucalyptus globulus*. It is very good at combating bacteria and viruses, making it a good disinfectant in cleaning the air during the ailment.

Cypress Oil

It is also known as *Cupresus semperivens*. This oil can make a perfect substitute for essential pine oil when used in cleaning.

Pine Oil

It is also known as *Pinus sylvestris*. It has a woody aroma. You can use this natural essential oil to improve your cleaning. It has analgesic, antiseptic, antimicrobial, and antispasmodic properties.

Peppermint Oil

It is also known as *Mentha piperita*. It is popularly known for its traditional medical uses and also culinary use. It is a great cleaning agent that blends well with other cleaning agents. It has a minty scent. It has analgesic, antiseptic, antimicrobial, and antispasmodic properties.

Spearmint Oil

It is also known as *Mentha spicata.* It is popularly used for cooking, and it has medicinal properties too. It is milder if you compare it with peppermint essential oil. It has analgesic, antiseptic, antimicrobial, and antispasmodic properties.

Geranium (Rose) Oil

It is also called *Pelargonium graveolons.* It is am oil that has is used to help prevent many health challenges. It can blend with many essential oil cleaning agents that are homemade.

Essential oils are usually concentrated, so for you to dilute them, you will need the help of base oil to make them less concentrated.

So I will be giving you the joint base oil you can use to dilute your essential oils.

There are different options out there when it comes to you using base oil. But I will suggest you use the one you are familiar with before digressing to use other ones.

So the standard oil I will be listing for you are; almond oil, apricot kernel, coconut oil, and jojoba oil.

Apricot Kernel Oil

Another name for It is *Prunus armeniaca*. It is gotten from the kernels of Apricots, by pressing. Even though it is perfect for the skin, it is used as a cleaning agent and as a carrier of other essential oils.

Almond Oil (Sweet)

This oil is also called *Prunus dulcis*. This oil is also good for your skin apart from it being an excellent cleaning oil for your home.

Note when getting Almond oil from your grocery store, make sure you get the ones that are sweet as others are bitter because of the production of cyanide by an enzyme when Almond oil mix with water. The colour is light gold.

Coconut Oil

Another name for this oil is *Cocos nucifera*. It is a perfect base for many household products. It is white and, at shallow temperatures, becomes tangible. This oil can be found in the market (both the refined and non-refined ones).

Jojoba Oil

It is also known as *Simmondsia chinensis*. This oil colour is bright golden and popularly known for its use in a skincare product. Although this oil is not used in cooking, it is used for cleaning home and serve as a good base for other essential oil.

The fourth formula is the choice of materials you will be needing in either making or preserving your green kitchen cleaner. So, let go ahead and discuss the standard equipment you will be needing.

1. Containers

After developing your homemade cleaning agents that are not harmful to the body, it is essential to know where to put them.

Often time's people put these things in a container that has been used to store cleaning suppliers. Even though you can use this container, I will not advise you to use it to store your new homemade cleaner. They might contaminate the substance inside it and thus reduce its effectiveness in cleaning your home appliances and other things you want to clean.

I would rather say you through away chemical containers and get new ones for new products or homemade chemicals.

But this doesn't mean that all of them are bad, like, for example, jars used to store food can be repurpose and use to store your homemade cleaners. Also, you can use jars free from microbial contaminants.

If you find it difficult getting what you will use to store your homemade cleaners, look around you, and you will be surprised by the number of containers you have at your disposer.

If you don't want any container at your home, you can also go and buy on for yourself. The price of the containers varies, so look around and get the one that is suitable for you are buying. One thing you have to know is that you don't need to spend much money to get these containers. The cheaper ones in the market will serve you.

When you get your container, make sure you label it appropriately to know which contains a particular supplier or the other.

2. Buckets

It will be needful to put your water and your cleaning agents before starting your cleaning.

3. paper towel

Paper towels are not recyclable that are affordable and easy to use for cleaning.

You can use it to dry your hand and surfaces. To make the utmost use of this, hang some in the sink and make sure you wash it every day to prevent the accumulation of germs. You can also place this in the kitchen to dry your hand

Alternatives to Paper Towel

An alternative to paper towel you can use to clean your environment is;

- **Non-Used Cloth Diapers:** You can use it as one or a new one. It has a high absorbent rate, so that makes it a good cleaner of a water spill.

- **Non-Used T-Shirts:** this can be used to mop up spills around the house. So you can look around and locate that t-shirt you are no more using and start making use of them.

- **Non-Used Towels and Washcloths:** if you have some old washcloths and towel you are not using, this can be perfect for cleaning messy places in your house.

4. Shop Towels

It can be called a commercial bar. They are heavy duty in nature. They are designed to clean up substances like grease.

Shop Towel Alternatives

The alternative of shop towel comes in various forms. So you have to locate one of your choice and use.

The beauty of these towels is that they are reusable when washed.

So this alternative range from flour sack towels, which is 100% cotton, thin, and lint-free and microfiber towels are absorbent and should not leave lint behind.

The next step in the formula is cleaning proper. This step is based on the fact that different ingredients are mixed to produce a green kitchen cleaner for a specific purpose. So, here we go with the steps.

Simple Cleaning

One of the vital things we need in life is good health, which comes to the proper cleanliness of our environment.

Every store in our environment has one cleaning product or the order that you can use to clean your environment. Still, I will like to recommend this 100% Natural Multi-purpose Cleaner for you to use.

In your quest to live a healthy lifestyle, your cabinets are usually filled with much commercial product that is harmful to the environment and health.

Cleanliness, which is also said to be hygiene, is a long topic that has existed since time immemorial. Our knowledge about hygiene and sanitation has grown, and we now know what to do always to keep yourself safes. In a developed country, it is reported that increment in life expectancy is attributed to regular personal hygiene and cleanliness.

Therefore this call for you taking it upon yourself to clean your environment at all cost and time.

The all-purpose cleaner works for everything, and it is a thing you can do for yourself.

Vinegar Spray

Task: replace the artificial cleaners you currently have. Get vinegar and water and mix it in the ratio of 1:1. It will form your all-purpose cleaning solution.

- Combine 1 cup white distilled vinegar with 1 cup of water
- Mix the two and put them in a spray bottle.

- Spray as desired any time you want to use. However, make sure you use it away from cloths.

Citrus Spray

- Combine 2 cup of white distilled vinegar with 1 cup of water
- Add 15–20 drops of lemon or orange citrus oils
- Mix the two and put them in a spray bottle.
- Spray as desired any time you want to use. However, make sure you use it away from cloths.

Amazing Multi-Purpose Cleaner

To make a fantastic multi-purpose cleaner, follow these steps

- Mix the following; 2 tablespoons white distilled vinegar, two teaspoon liquid castile soap, four tablespoons baking soda, and 4 cups warm water.
- Combine the first three ingredients, then wait for

> the vinegar and baking
> soda to stop reacting.
> - Afterwards, add the warm
>   water and shake gently to
>   mix well.

You can make it anytime you need to clean .surfaces and disinfect.

Multi-purpose disinfectant

For a long natural multi-purpose spray is used by various folks to disinfect their environment against micro-organism.

History has it that during the bubonic plague outbreak in the middle age, robbers that stole from the plague victims in a French town of Marseilles prevented themselves from contacting the plague with a magic essential oil which is garlic, eucalyptus, lemon, rosemary, and sage by washing themselves with the liquid.

It has survived throughout history because of its effectiveness. It is referred to as thieves oil blend.

Primary Ingredients for Thieves Oil Blend

The primary ingredients are 40 drops of clove bud essential oil, 35 drops lemon essential oil, 20 drops cinnamon bark essential oil, 15 drops eucalyptus essential oil, and ten drops rosemary essential oil.
Make sure you add all the essential oils in a dark glass container. Let the lid of the container close tightly, then shake to mix all oils well.

Making of Thieves Oil Disinfectant Spray

To make the thieves oil disinfectant spray, you have to combine the following;

- 2 cup of water
- 16–20 drops Thieves Oil Blend
- Add water and Thieves Oil Blend using a spray bottle.

Note: Before each use, makes sure you shake It very well. So, you spray it on the surface or the air any time you need to disinfect your environment.

Lemon-Lime Dust Spray

Another organic spray that is very good in cleaning your home is the lemon-lime dust spray.

To make a cloud of lemon-lime dust spray, you have to mix the following substances;

- ½ of cup lemon juice
- 1/2 cup water
- Ten drops of lime essential oil
- Ten drops of lemon essential oil

You have to mix all this component in a spray bottle and shake well.

You spray on dusty surfaces and using a clean cloth you wipe away.

To avoid the solution from spoiling due to the presence of lemon juice, you can put the remnant of the solution into a refrigerator.

In any case, you have dirty and dusty surfaces, you can use cedar dust soap to clean the surfaces;

Forming a Cedar Dust Soap Solution

To form a Cedar Dust Soap Solution, you have to mix the following;

- 1/2 cup of castile soap
- 3/2 cup of water
- 40 drops of cedar oil

You can put all the solution in a spray bottle after mixing well. Spray it onto a surface and clean with a clean cloth.

Make sure you shake very well before any use.

One of the properties bleach usually have is its ability to disinfect an environment. But that doesn't guarantee its safety. Some of the chemicals used to make this bleach are not organic but somewhat artificial, which may have a secondary effect on the body.

It is said that bleach can kill many strains of bacteria and viruses. But the disadvantage is that it can cause some health effect that is negative to human survival.

The question now is, is there any alternative to bleach that we can use to clean our environment and won't affect our health?

Keep reading!!

All-Purpose Vinegar And Hydrogen Disinfectant Spray

The substitute for bleach is All-Purpose vinegar and hydrogen disinfectant spray.

In Virginia Polytechnic Institute and State University, Dr Susan Sumner revealed that using white distilled vinegar solution in combination with hydrogen peroxide can destroy dreadful viruses and bacterial even better than bleach prepared artificially, and this does not affect the body.

So, all you need to do is to clean your environment with 50 % vinegar solution, you can either spray, or you use the scrub. After that, you clean the surface again with hydrogen peroxide, which can be sprayed or scrubbed.

Make sure you don't mix the solution; instead, you use them one after the other.

When vinegar is mixed with hydrogen peroxide, it forms peroxyacetic acid, also known as peracetic acid. Peroxyacetic acid is a potent oxidizing agent and can cause many of the same problems associated with bleach.

Home Made Disinfecting Wipes

Using a readymade cleaning wipe can be easy, but there a lot of non -organic ones out there which are not suitable for the health and can be harmful to the body.

I recommend you go with this **100% Natural Multi-purpose Cleaner** or you make your natural wipes yourself using the in this book as will be given to you as we progress.

- Mix 2 cup of water with
- Four tablespoons of white distilled vinegar and
- Four tablespoons of castile soap
- 40 drops of any of the following essential oils (mix and match!): Thieves Oil Blend (24), thyme, tea tree, lemon, lavender, or rosemary

Note: the ingredient should be mixed and put in an airtight container with a ball of cotton wool and store in a dark room that is cooled.

Make sure you shake very well before using them.

Change your Clorox wipes with homemade disinfecting wipes by putting cloth wipes and homemade disinfecting solution in a glass jar.

The last secret is ways to clean the kitchen using the green cleaner for a significant result. So as you continue in this part, you should be able to use the green cleaner you made yourself clean your kitchen for effective leaving.

The last secret

You must have known that the kitchen is one of the significant parts of the house that can be filled with germs because of the unique home activities that go on there.

A study has revealed, there is much number of faecal bacteria in sink handles found in the kitchen than we can find anywhere in the bathroom.

Also, various surfaces in the kitchen like sponges and dishcloths, faucet handles, cutting boards, and the sink are the primary place we can find bacteria grow and spread exponentially from one person to another.

So for you to start cleaning your kitchen more hygienically, you can either use the 100% **Natural Multi-purpose Cleaner** or make use natural cleaner as explained in this book by creating one for yourself and positioning them in sinks, countertops, and appliances.

Thus cleaners are the All-Purpose vinegar and hydrogen disinfectant spray; Citrus Spray will serve very well. However, the thieves Oil Blend Disinfectant Spray is the best for kitchen cleaning.

Another recipe that can be very useful in cleaning your kitchen is wood, stone, or stainless steel; continue reading.

Food Prep: Cutting Boards

You need to use the cotton board in the kitchen as this helps to keep bacteria localize in a particular area of your kitchen

Much contamination in the kitchen is found in the cutting board.

Raw meats have much contamination of bacteria more when compared with vegetables, fruit, or bread. Thus, much care should be taken when preparing and cooking meat.

If you are making a variety of foods, the best way to do It is to have many cutting boards: which includes;

- 1 for meat,
- 1 for your produce
- 1 for bread

However, if you have butcher block counters in the kitchen for food every preparation, I recommend you have at least one cutting board that you can remove exclusively, and for raw meats, you can wash them in the sink.

Bacteria can get lodged in tiny cuts and nicks in plastic and into the grain of the wood, which is porous. However, wood cutting boards have the ability to lodges more bacteria when compared to nonporous plastic. On the other hand, plastic boards can move quickly than wood boards.

But, for nonporous cutting board materials, like pyro ceramic and glass, no much research has been done. It might be because those materials are hard on knives. Thus are not used by people as when compared to the plastic and wood cotton board.

Various types of cutting boards possess unique benefits. Naturally, woods are biodegradable and have anti-bacterial properties, and it is less expensive than plastic.

BPA-free plastic cutting boards are often thinner, making it easier to have multiple cutting boards in a small kitchen and prevent the spread of bacteria. Irrespective of the cutting boards you are using in your kitchen, it is necessary to wash them very well to kill any bacteria lingering around the cutting board.

Cleaning Plastic Cutting Boards

You can wash plastic cutting boards in a dish. Still, research shows that bacteria can transfer from cutting board can be transferred to other dishes in the dishwasher.

Therefore the safest way to clean plastic board is scrub using boiling and soapy water.

If you want extra protection, spray the cutting board with vinegar and wiping it with a clean cloth after washing.

Cleaning Wood Cutting Boards and Butcher Block Counters

To clean wood cutting board;

- Put the board in hot and soapy water.
- Use a bristle brush to scrub
- Rinse it and allow it to dry.

To clean butcher block countertops;

- Scrub using hot and soapy water.
- Brush or sponge the catcher block.

However, for light cleaning of butcher block;

- Spray using vinegar.
- Wipe with a clean cloth.
- Dry your cutting board and butcher block thoroughly after cleaning them.

Note that wet wood is a suitable environment for the growth of bacteria, resulting in secondary health consequences.

Don't add wood cutting boards in the dishwasher, and don't brush made of wires on wood cutting boards or butcher block. These can cause severe damage to the boards.

Special Butcher Block And Wood Cutting Board Cleaner

We will be looking at some special cleaner we can use to clean butcher block and wood cutting board to yield maximum cleaning results.

Salt And Lemon Butcher Block And Wood Cutting Board Cleaner

Apart from the use of hot and soapy water to clean the woody cutting board. You can also make use of; coarse salt and Lemon juice

For a deeper cleaning of your butcher block and wood cutting board;

- Sprinkle coarse salt liberally on the board.
- Squeeze the juice from two lemons on the board
- Scrub for some minutes using a bristle brush.
- Finally, rinse and dry.

The acid in the citrus fruits will help kill much of the bacteria lodging on the butcher block.

If you need a different citrus smell, you scrub with a lime or orange juice.

Baking Soda And Vinegar Butcher Block And Wood Cutting Board Cleaner

Apart from using hot and soapy water to clean the woody cutting board, you can also make use of; baking soda and distilled white vinegar.

An alternative to of salt and lemon, you can do the following;

- Spray baking soda on the board.

- Include a couple of tablespoons of vinegar.

- Using a bristle brush, scrub for several minutes.

- Rinse and allow to dry.

Note: You can also use salt and vinegar or baking soda and lemon. The salt and baking soda serve as abrasives, which aid loosen grime and lift it away; white vinegar and lemon possess anti-bacterial properties that aid kill bacteria and combat odours.

Counters

Either in the bathroom or kitchen, counters are places bacteria always like to stay. To reduce the growth of bacterial, all kitchen surfaces have to be cleaned after preparing food.

All kitchen surfaces can be cleaned well using a good scrub, soap, and hot water.

However, for solid surface counters, you can decide to use any of the all-purpose recipes.

I will unleash more recipe ideas for some of the most popular (nonplastic) counter materials as we continue.

Wood Counter

You can use wood butcher block counters as cutting surfaces, just like other wood cutting surfaces. The wood has to be cleaned thoroughly to avoid bacteria growth and be treated using natural oils instead of artificial petroleum- or polyurethane-based products.

A user makes typically use of mineral oil to treat butcher block. Still, this oil is gotten from petroleum, thus not biodegradable, nor is it the best choice.

The same goes for paraffin wax. While not try all-natural oils to condition your wood rather than using synthetic oil.

Robin Wood, an internationally respected woodworker with twenty years of woodworking experience, revealed that oils are good stand s as a good wine in the industry.

Robin Wood makes use of oils grown close to him, which are "safe enough to drink." He makes use of walnut and linseed oils, which are both natural, and he is also comfortable using tung oil, which serves as a replacement for mineral oil.

Tung oil is gotten from flaxseed. All these oils are natural and can be used in food preparation.

Using Linseed oil has a colour that can give wood a yellow hue after use with time. So while buying linseed oil, don't purchase boiled linseed oil that possesses chemical driers.

In other to avoid additives in this oil, buy raw, pure oil. You can get walnut oil in any grocery store's oils section.

You can buy Tung and linseed oils online or in any local pharmacy or craft store. Note that the oil to be should be a pure oil without additive.

Caution: oils left on rags get caught up by the fire. Many fire outbreaks have resulted in this, so caution should be taking to avoid such from happening.

Make sure you remove toxins present in counters: Treat butcher block counters using pure coconut or walnut oil.

Coconut oil is another food-safe oil that can be used on counters. It is challenging to get rancid, and it is very stable. However, what I like about wood is if you use what is not right on it, you can sand it out using sandpaper.

Every month make sure you oil your butcher block counters, and that is if they are old, but if they are new, you do that weekly.

How to Use Your Natural Oil

- To use your natural oil, position the bottle containing the oil in hot water for some minute to warm it.
- Put some quantity on the wood.
- Using a soft cloth distributes the oil evenly.
- Allow the oil to sit overnight and to use a clean cloth, wipe off any excess oil.

Stone

Some counters are made naturally with stones. They are a common choice for kitchens. Examples of everyday stone use are granite, marble, quartz, slate, and travertine are just a few of the many possibilities.

The rule for stones counter

- In case of any spill, wipe immediately.
- Don't use Acidic cleaner and sandpaper entirely.

- Don't place hot object directly on the holder. You can use a potholder, trivet, or any holder available within your reach.

Some stone counter is engineered made using quartz and a binder. It can scratch and heat resistant when compared with natural stone.

Treat every stone counter with care, irrespective of their make.

- For light cleaning, you can use a Heavy-Duty Glass Cleaner bottle close on hand, and this applies to natural and engineered stone counters.
- A clean cloth can be used to spray cleaner on the counter.
- You can use soap and boiling water for more massive cleaning, or you can use any of the recipes we will be given below.

Coconut Oil Counter Rub

Some counters are porous.

These counters are attended to especially.

These include granite and butcher block.

These counters do better when they are treated weekly. The best and easy way to treat this counter is to rub with coconut oil, which is naturally antimicrobial, anti-bacterial, antiviral, and antifungal.

The oil has a low melting point, so the season of the environment matters while using your coconut oil as they will be either a liquid or a solid.

Either of the two, all you need is a little of the oil to rub into the counter.

You allow the oil to soak into the pore of the counter, and you will verify this by noticing lines appearing on the counter.

To buff it, you use a clean, dry cloth.

Your counter will be free from every micro-organism after doing this process of cleaning the counter with coconut oil.

Granite Counter Cleaner

When it comes to the cleaning of granite counter, you make the following together to form a solution;

- 1 cup of vodka
- 2 cup of water
- Two drops of dish soap
- A few drops of essential oil of choice
- Use a small spray bottle to mix all components and shake well before you use them.

The solution will be used to clean granite anytime you wish to clean your counter made of granite.

Marble

Marble is formed when limestone is heated or pressured. It is in a class of soft rock and is made up predominantly of calcium carbonate.

It can be damaged easily by acidic substances. Therefore, don't use vinegar or lemon juice to clean marble! Instead, use soap and water for ordinary cleaning.

In case of organic stain like coffee, wine, and so on from marble, to use the following recipe, a trick that the United States government uses to clean historical marble statues.

And that is the use of marble stone stain remover.

Marble Stain Remover

This stain remover consists of;

- Hydrogen peroxide

- A white absorbent material: which can be crushed white chalk, unbleached white flour, or white paper towels

So the process involved in the removing of the stains are as follows;

- Clean the stained area with water.
- Using hydrogen peroxide wet the area.
- Mix enough hydrogen peroxide with the absorbent material to create a poultice or paste.
- I am using the poultice to apply the thick layer on and around the stain.
- Using pieces of plastic, cover the poultice, and use tape to secure it.
- Allow a poultice to sit for 48 hours.
- Moisten it using water and use a spatula to remove.

Metal

Countertops are usually made of metals, which include stainless steel, zinc, pewter, copper, and bronze, which are attractive options for kitchens.

They last long and don't need finishes or seal. Some of these metals resist heat and stain. Some have nice patina if you do not polish them regularly, and others are recyclable.

Copper and copper-containing alloys are one of the best choices because copper is anti-bacterial naturally.

The research revealed that bacterial like E. coli bacteria died when placed on the surface of copper for 90 minutes when refrigerated or 270 minutes at room temperature. A similar result was also discovered when the test was conducted on the influenza virus.

Stainless Steel Counter Cleaner

Formation of a stainless steel cleaner is;

- 2 part cream of tartar
- 2 part hydrogen peroxide

The procedure involved in the cleaning is;

- Mix cream of tartar and hydrogen peroxide into a paste.
- Apply to counter.
- Wipe off with a damp cloth.
- Buff with a clean and dry cloth for extra shine.

Copper Counter Cleaner

The primary ingredient for a copper counter cleaner is one lemon and coarse salt.

To clean metal surfaces with the copper counter cleaner, perform the following;

- Cut a lemon in half.

- Sprinkle it with coarse salt.
- Rub over the copper counter
- Wipe with a damp cloth.

More Common Counter Choices

There are also other choices of cleaners for the kitchen counter we will discuss. One of such standard counter is the ceramic tiles.

Ceramic tile has some sort of style and colour it gives to the kitchen. Some of these tiles are mixed with lead, and as such, you must cover tile occasionally to avoid mildew and stains.

Like stone, ceramic tile can be damaged by acid, so avoid using vinegar- or lemon-based cleaners on them.

Another material is porcelain, which is a traditional material counter found in the bathroom.
They are durable and easy to clean. To clean it, you can make use of a non-acidic scrub or disinfecting recipes

made for the bathroom. We will be discussing it as we proceed.

Ceramic, Tile, And Porcelain Counter Cleaner

To clean Ceramic, Tile, And Porcelain Counter, we can make use of a Heavy-Duty Glass Cleaner.

You can make it by mixing;

- 20–40 total drops of essential oils. Preferable from the one or more from the Thieves Oil Blend,
- Add thyme oil
- Add tea tree oil
- Put the Heavy-Duty Glass Cleaner in a spray bottle
- Include the essential oil
- Shake all the mixture very well.

Cleaner Boosters

The boosters of basic cleaner are Thieves Oil Blend, thyme oil, and tea tree oil. This booster is majorly in their anti-bacterial capability.

Kitchen Sinks

Areas prone to moisture, like sinks and dish cleaning tools, are easily exposed to bacterial growth and transfer.

To keep the sink clean and healthy, you have to;

- Keeping these areas dry will help slow the growth of bacteria
- Keeping a basket of towels under your sink
- Wipe sink and counters down using a clean and dry cloth.
- Toss the towel and the dishcloth into the laundry.

Do the following a few days later,

- Scrub and raise you the sink's drain catcher.

- Keep the sink clean by boiling and do the same for others.

- Use any of the sink recipes we will explain as we progress to scrub your sink.

- After all,, rinse with hot water.

Sink Essentials

The Essential Sink Cleaner is suitable for cleaning stainless steel and sinks made up of porcelain. Make use of cloths that is soft in combination with sponges or bristle brushes that is soft to clean stainless steel sinks to avoid harming the finish.

Essential Sink Cleaner

Essential sink cleaner is made up of the following;

- 1 cup of white distilled vinegar

- ½ cup of baking soda

- Ten drops of any essential oil of your choice.

When you are done with your cleaning, you can wipe down the remaining debris with water, and after that, wet the sink using vinegar.

The baking soda can be sprinkled on it and a few drops of any essential oil of your choice.
While scrubbing the sink using the cloth, a form paste will be formed by the baking soda and vinegar.

When you are done, rinse with water thoroughly.

Sweet Cinnamon Sink Scrub

Sanitize the dirtiest area of your house kitchen sink using Sweet Cinnamon Sink Scrub. Combine baking soda, cinnamon, and sweet orange essential oil to destroy bacteria and germs.

It is one among the sink scrub that smells good, and you can use it anytime you feel like.

It is formed by combining the following ingredient;

- 2 cup of baking soda

- Two tablespoon of ground cinnamon
- Ten drops of sweet orange essential oil

Combine every ingredient in a container that is airtight.

To use it, spray part of the sweet Cinnamon Sink cleaner on a wet sink.

You can use a cloth scrub to clean, and afterward,s you rinse using clean water.

Scrubber for Sink Stain

To form a sink stain scrubber, mix the following as outlined below;

- 1 cup of borax
- 1 cup of baking soda
- 20–30 drops of tea tree essential oil

Make sure that all these ingredients are mixed in an airtight container.

To clean the sink,

- Sprinkle on the stained area,

- Scrub using a damp cloth.

- Apply vinegar to rinse.

- Then after that, use hot water to rinse.

Super Lemon Stain Remover

To form super lemon stain remover, you have to combine the ingredient that will be listed below;

- 1 cup of baking soda
- 20 drops of lemon oil

Make sure that all these ingredients are mixed to form a paste.

To clean the sink,

- Apply on the stain areas
- Allow the mixture to stay for a few hours or overnight.
- Scrub gently the spot

- Rinse very well using water.

Clogged Sink Cleaner

What happens when you have clogged drains?

Do the following to clean;

- Don't use aromatic chemicals, which can cause illness and destroy your pipes.
- You can make use of baking soda and vinegar as they will aid in unclogging the blocked pipe.
- Using boiling water will aid in loosening and flushing the debris away.

Get the following ingredient;

- 1 cup of baking soda
- 2 cup of vinegar
- 2 gallon of boiling water

Using the mixture, clean your clogged pipe through the following steps;

- Put the baking soda into the drain

- Apply vinegar

- Allow to bubble and react for 30 to 40 minutes.

- Boil at least 2 gallons of water

- Flush the drain with the boiling water.

- Repeat if necessary.

To clean your kitchen garbage disposals, you can apply the following steps;

- **Run cold water when using your disposal.**

Doing this will help grease that moves through the drain to become solidify while get chopped up by the disposal. Using hot water might result in grease liquefying, which will result in a grease pool in the pipes, resulting in clogs and foul odours.

- **Run Your Garbage Disposal Regularly.**

Allowing it to run for long can cause accumulation of rust. Thus, causing your disposal useless.

- **Don't be Hard.**

The disposal is to help you deal with those food scraps that made its way into the sink. Items that are not food, large items, and food particles that are large can be disposed of properly in the garbage or compost.

- **Allow water to run.**

When you have a running garbage disposal, water can also be running in it. Allow water to run continually for at least 15 seconds when you are done turning off. It will help the disposal to stop the formation of small particles, which will potentially clog the disposal while rotting food will result in to smell you won't want in your kitchen.

Icy Cold Disposal Cleaner

This consist of the following;

- A handful of ice cubes
- 1-2 cup regular or rock salt

The dispose of the garbage, you do the following;

- Toss the ice cubes and salt into your garbage disposal.
- Allow sitting for a few minutes
- Put on the cold water
- Run the disposal until all the ice breaks down and finally disappears.
- The ice chips will scour your disposal, cleaning away grime.

You can also use vinegar to run the garbage disposal through the following steps;

- Allow the vinegar to freeze into cube trays.
- Add a handful of vinegar ice cubes into the drain

- Add 2 cups of baking soda.

- Allow cold water to run into the disposal

- Turn on all the disposal until all the ice breaks down and finally disappears.

- The ice chips will scour the disposal while baking soda and vinegar help in cleaning away odours.

Natural Disposal Scourer

To form a natural disposal scourer, you make use of eggshells.

Broken eggshells create particles that help wash the sides of the disposal because of its abrasive nature.

Citrus Peel Disposal Cleaner

To prepare a citrus peel disposal cleaner;

- Take 3 or 4 oranges, lemons, or limes that are about to go wrong.
- Cut into two halves and put them, one at a time, into the disposal.
- Make sure cold water is running while doing this.
- Put on the disposal.
- Allow the disposal chop each half, rind and all.
- The rinds will aid scour away grime, and the citrus oils will aid combat odours.

Baking Soda Disposal Deodorizer

To form a baking soda disposal deodorizer, mix the following;

- Add 2 cups of baking soda into the disposal.
- Allow it to settle for at least 1 hour.
- Add 2–4 cups of vinegar into the disposal
- Run the disposal while the vinegar bubbles.

Borax Disposal Deodorizer

To prepare borax disposal;

- Add eight tablespoons of borax into the disposal.
- Allow settling for 2 hours.
- Add hot water, vinegar, or both.

The majority of the bacteria found in the kitchen comes from food. The bacteria is transferred during cutting or preparation of food and during mess clean up.

Bacteria can move from raw meat, cutting board, to washing sponge, to the handle of the sink, to the next person hands who use the sink, another area that the person may likely touch.

To reduce the spread of bacteria, carefully clean the food preparation surfaces, utensils thoroughly using soap and hot water after using it.

You can get this already prepared 100% Natural Multi-purpose Cleaner or make use of a 2:20 ratio of castile soap and water.

Add it in a squirt bottle, and using your sponge or scrub brush, clean the utensil or area you intend to clean.

You can decide to use vinegar water rinse to clean your dishes. You may even discover a thin film on your dishes.

The thin film comes from salts that remain after castile soap reacts with minerals in the water, which is a significant problem if the water you are using is problematic.

Using Vinegar help remove the salts. When you are done rinsing the soapy dishes off with water, using another rinse bucket with a quart of water and a cup of vinegar ready.

When you are done cleaning, place the dish on a rack.

Apart from dunking your dishes in vinegar, you can decide to spray your dish using vinegar-and-water mixture on the drying rack.

However, it is not a wise decision to put vinegar (an acid) directly to soap (a base) and water, since they will react chemically together.

However, if do want to use a Castile wash or already made **100% Natural Multi-purpose Cleaner** you can try essential dish soap by trying to mix the following;

- 1/2 cup of tightly packed, grated bar soap
- ½ cups of boiling water
- Two tablespoon of washing soda
- ½ cup of castile soap
- 40–60 total drops of your chosen essential oils

To form the essential dish soap;

- Put in grated soap to the boiling water.
- Stir until dissolved.
- Put in washing soda and castile soap.
- Stir very well and remove from heat.
- Make the combination to cool
- Put in essential oils.
- Store in a glass jar or soap dispenser.

Simple Citrus Dish Soap

Another dish soap you can use is the simple citrus dish soap formed by the following ingredients;

- 40 ounces of castile soap
- 40 drops of lime or lemon essential oil
- 40 drops of sweet orange essential oil

Combine all ingredients. And use whenever you want to wash your dish.

Floral Dish Soap

Another dish soap you can use is the floral dish soap formed by the following ingredients;

- 40 ounces of castile soap
- 20 drops of lavender oil
- 20 drops of ylang-ylang oil
- 20 drops of rosemary oil

Combine all ingredients. And use whenever you want to wash your dish.

Dish Washing Tools

Making use of sponges that have deep holes which can trap food particles and has a high damp tendency forms reasonable breeding grounds for bacteria.

The majority of commercial sponges are manufactured from petroleum derivatives, which are not suitable for the environment.

The following are few alternatives to such sponge available through several online retailers, which will help you cut down bacterial growth.

Hemp Scrubbers

Generally, It is more abrasive when compared to cotton; however, it is soft enough for every regular dishwashing needs.

Between uses, make sure you hang hemp scrubber to dry, at one or two-day interval, throw them in the laundry.

Cotton Dishcloths

You can get dishcloths from the market that have some texture to them, or you can also knit your own if you have the skill.

After every use, hang to allow it dry, and everyone or two-day interval launder.

Coconut Scrubbers

You can use coconut coir fibre to make different scrubbers and pads made from the husks of coconuts.

Coconut fibre is biodegradable and can form an excellent cleaner scrub.

Make sure you disinfect regularly.

Loofah Scrubbers

Loofahs are gotten from gourds. Therefore they are biodegradable. However, they can trap bacteria.

To prevent trapping of bacteria, dry after every use.
Sterilize them at least once a week.
When you are done using them, compost the material.

Sponges

Some of you might prefer sponge to the other scrubber described above. So, I will prefer you to go for biodegradable cellulose sponges. They immediately start showing signs of wear, please replace them.

Researchers discovered high concentrations of bacteria in kitchen surfaces in a home that don't change their sponge regularly.

Make sure dishcloths, sponges, and scrub brushes are kept in a location like a hanger where they can quickly get dry by sunshine.

You can sterilize them by putting them into a pot of boiling water and staying for 15 minutes, after that dry.

You can also put your sponge in the dishwasher for a full wash and dry cycle, or wash your dishcloths in the washing machine. While washing,, you can put in vinegar or tea tree oil to the rinse cycle.

Dishwashers

It is reported that washing dishes using an automatic dishwasher is more effective than using hand to wash them.

Based on the instruction from dishwasher manufacturers, It is how to wash dishes in the dishwasher:

- Don't Rinse Dishes. What to do is, scrape food particles into a trash can.
- Wash a complete set of dishes to maximize water and energy use for washing.
- Make use of available energy-saving features in the Automatic Dishwasher.

However, less energy can be consumed by you washing your dishes manually instead of using automatic, and that is if you are washing a dish at one time.

Wash in a bowl and rinse in another bowl.

However, in case you don't have an automatic dishwasher, you can use the following recipes to keep your dishes and dishwasher clean:

Simple Dishwasher Detergent

You can form your simple dishwasher detergent by using the ingredient;

- 2 cup of borax
- 2 cup of washing soda
- 1 cup of kosher salt
- 1 cup of citric acid

Combine all the ingredients. Make sure you are careful not to inhale as you mix. Use two tablespoons of detergent per load. And preserve in an airtight container.

Lemon-Powered Dishwasher Detergent

You can form your Lemon-Powered dishwasher detergent by using the ingredient;

- 2 cups of borax

- 4 cups of baking soda

- 2 cup of citric acid

- 40–60 drops of lemon essential oil

Combine all the ingredients. Make sure you are careful not to inhale as you mix. Use two tablespoons of detergent per load. And preserve in an airtight container.

Lavender Dishwasher Detergent

You can form your lavender dishwasher detergent by using the ingredient;

- 2 cups of washing soda

- 2 cup of borax

- 2 cup of baking soda

- 40–60 drops lavender oil

Combine all the ingredients. Make sure you are careful not to inhale as you mix. Use two tablespoons of detergent per load. And preserve in an airtight container.

Dishwasher Gel

You can form your lavender dishwasher detergent by using the ingredient;

- 2 cups of water
- ½ cup of soap flakes or grated bar soap
- Two tablespoons of glycerin
- Four tablespoons of white distilled vinegar

Combine all the ingredients in a saucepan and allow to a boil over medium heat. When all the soap has dissolved, remove from heat and keep to cool completely. Store in an airtight container and use two tablespoons per load.

Lemon Dishwasher Gel

You can form your lavender dishwasher detergent by using the ingredient;

- 4 cups of castile soap
- 1 cup of water
- 1 cup of lemon juice
- 40 drops of lemon essential oil

Combine all ingredients using a saucepan over medium-high heat. Make sure you stir to make sure all the ingredients are dissolved. Allow to cool and store in an airtight container and use two tablespoons per load.

Simple Spot Remover

Sometimes you may have clean dishes, but when spots plague the glass wash in the dishwasher, you can decide to get a commercial spot remover.

The good news is this; you don't need to get a commercial spot remover because provision will be made for that as we proceed in this book.

The solution to spot Remover

Do the following to make a dishwasher spot remover;

- Put a diluted vinegar solution to the rinse aid compartment. Make sure the rinse takes care of the spots.
- Add six parts of white distilled vinegar
- Add 2 part of the water

After the above mixture, dilute vinegar using water and add it rinse aid compartment. Run dishwasher as usual.

You can also choose to use straight vinegar in the dishwasher as a rinse aid. It is based on your decision anyway.

Nevertheless, 100% vinegar can render your dishes spot-free; the high acidic content of vinegar can damage the rubber and plastic in the rinse aid compartment. To prevent this from happening, dilute the vinegar to avoid this risk.

Vinegar Dishwasher Deep Cleaner

Sometime dishwasher will need to be cleaned deeply as some food particles can be collected in it. This may start to smell, which not an acceptable form of hygiene.

To prevent this,

- Put two mugs with white distilled vinegar in the dishwasher
- Put on the top rack and one on the bottom, with the mugs sitting upright.
- Put on your dishwasher as usual.

- As water pours into the mugs, the vinegar will slowly clean your dishwasher.

Lemonade Dishwasher Deep Cleaner

You can use the Lemonade Dishwasher Deep Cleaner by following the steps below;

- Add a few packets of lemon-flavoured drink mix (such as Kool-Aid) into your dishwasher.
- Run the cycle as usual.
- The citric acid in the drink mix will aid in cleaning the dishwasher.

Pots And Pans

The majority of the pots and pans used in the kitchen are made with a nonstick (Teflon) coating, which is not suitable for the health of humans.

The Teflon coating reduces burning and makes cooking and cleaning easy. But when the coating reaches a specific temperature, the toxic and carcinogenic substance is released, and this, on the other hand, affects the health of humans.

To avoid this, you will be considering using this alternative cooking pots or pans.

Cast Iron

Using a pot or a pan coated with cast iron is a suitable medium of cooking.

It is economical to buy and use; it efficiently absorbs and distributes heat. Evenly.

Cast iron can last for decades.

Cast iron is porous, having in porous holes in its surface. Before use, make sure you season cast iron cookware to prevent your food from burning and sticking and also from rusting.

During seasoning, brand new cast iron, clean it using soap, hot water, and a stiff (not wire) scrub brush and dry it thoroughly.

You can either use a soft cloth or paper towel to spread lard or vegetable oil all over the inside surface.

Bake the pot upside down on a cookie sheet for 1 hour at 350 degrees Fahrenheit.

Because of the presence of oil on the pot, you will notice smoke in the air; turn on your exhaust fan and open a window.

Anytime you use your cast iron, it will become more seasoned. In the end, you will see a shiny black patina.

Cleaning Cast Iron

After using your cast iron, scrape excess food off with a spoon or a scrub brush (not a wire scrub brush), first without water, and then with hot water running over the pan. If food is stuck on, pour boiling water into the pan. Let it sit and soften the food for a few minutes. Pour it out and scrape again.

Another trick you can try for stuck-on food is scrub the cast iron with coarse table salt and a soft cloth before rinsing it with water. If you use soap and water, you will need to season the cast iron. Water and scraping alone should be enough to clean your cast iron.

Place the pan on a hot stove burner or in the oven for a few minutes to dry it thoroughly. Once it is dry and cool, put another thin layer of oil or lard on it, removing any excess with a soft cloth or paper towel.

Do not put cast iron in an automatic dishwasher, as this can remove the seasoned coating and cause rust to form.

Storing Cast Iron

To store cast iron in a dry place.

Allow a soft cloth or paper towel—this aids in absorbing excess moisture.

Enameled Cast Iron

It is cast iron, which is covered by a thin layer of enamel.

Its properties are safe to cook food with it, it is durable, and you can use it without seasoning it.

Since you don't season it, it can be cleaned using soap and water.

Copper

Most professional chefs like copper pots or pans because of their property of conducting heat very well.

It is a highly reactive metal. Thus, it can react with some selected foods like tomatoes and other foods that are acidic. Therefore anyone who ingests such food cooked with cooper food becomes ill.

To avoid this, make use of copper cookware lined with stainless steel.

You can wash copper cookware with soap and water.

You can use a Copper Counter Cleaner when the copper pot or pan becomes stained, or you can make a paste from a lemon juice and baking soda. Use to paste to rub on the copper, then clean using a clean, dry, soft cloth before using washing with soap and water.

Stainless Steel and Anodized Aluminum

We still have other cookware that is made of stainless steel and anodized aluminium. These materials are durable and don't react with acidic or alkaline foods. They are also cheaper than copper or cast iron.

Stainless steel cookware has other metals, mostly copper or aluminium, that helps it to conduct heat evenly.

Heating your stainless steel cookware's first by adding a small amount of cooking oil before doing your everyday cooking helps prevent the sticking of food on the stainless steel.

You might ask yourself, what is Anodized aluminium?

In a layman word, it is processed aluminium; it has a nonreactive coating. It isn't porous. Therefore there is no need for adding oil to prevent food from sticking to the cookware. Instead, you should preheat the Anodized aluminium pot to help cook the food evenly.

KEYNOTE: Research has revealed a relationship between aluminium and Alzheimer's disease. For this reason, we recommend any scratched anodized aluminium cookware should be replaced immediately to avoid food from coming in contact with the aluminium surface.

Use soap and water to clean stainless steel and anodized aluminium cookware. In case there is burned food on the cookware that will be difficult to come out of the pot through your regular washing, do the following to clean;

- Boil water in the pan for 10–20 minutes to loosen the food
- Allow the pan cool
- Wash the cookware with your soap and water again.

Or alternatively,

- Put a tablespoon or two of baking soda into the
  pan
- Put enough water to create a paste.
- Scrub the pan with a sponge or soft brush.

General Rule: Avoid pouring cold water into a hot cookware's, as this can cause warping in cookware. Therefore, to pour water, leave pans to cool before washing to protect your health and the pan.

The majority of fruits and vegetables people sell in the market are full of pesticides. It is something you wouldn't want to eat. To remove this pesticide, you can try this inexpensive pesticide remover from the surfaces of your food.

The Dirty Dozen Plus And The Clean Fifteen

To stay away from chemicals in food, organic options are the best way to do that, but they are more expensive.

Therefore you have to choose wisely by stretching your budget. You can go online to look at the "Dirty Dozen Plus", and the "Clean Fifteen" lists released by the Environmental Working Group (EWG).

This list is not constant, as it is updated every year. The top twelve vegetables likely affected by pesticides are found in The Dirty Dozen. These are the vegetable or fruits you take note of.

To check the list of fruits and vegetables easily affected by pesticides, you can check the Clean Fifteen. Therefore, to save money, purchase the conventionally (non-organically) grown versions of your vegetable and fruits.

Vinegar Vegetable Spray

To clean hard-skinned vegetables and fruits, do the following;

- Getaway with spraying the food
- Allow it to settle for a few seconds
- Gently scrub the vegetable or fruits in clean, freshwater.
- Finally, use All-Purpose Vinegar Spray to aid cutting through the pesticides.

Alternatively;

- Put or scrub fruits and vegetables gently using All-Purpose Vinegar Spray
- Rinse using water to cut through pesticides used on conventional produce.

Vinegar Fruit Soak

If the vegetable is soft to clean, following the steps outlined below;

- Soak the vegetable instead of scrubbing.
- Combine your 1:1 vinegar-and-water solution, and allow the vegetable to soak for a minute or two.
- After that, rinse everything off using fresh water.

Cleaning the Refrigerator

When food spills, you can clean it up quickly, but sometimes you might not have the time or be at home to clean any food spills.

To avoid the above from happening, you have to try the following steps to make sure your refrigerator is clean;

Of course, you know that nothing messes up the refrigerator like rotting, mouldy foods.
So, what are these steps?

Lemon Fridge Spritz

To form a lemon fridge sprit;

- Try combining a 1:1 solution of water and lemon juice.
- The lemon juice will kill bacteria because of its acidic nature while giving the fridge a refreshing scent.

To clean the around the refrigerator, gaskets and doors.
- Take the lemon spritz and an old toothbrush and clean out these hard-to-reach areas.

Citrus Fridge Deodorizer

To prepare a citrus fridge deodorizer, sue the following ingredient;

- Two small box of baking soda
- 40–60 total drops of citrus essential oil (try lemon, orange, lime, or grapefruit)
- Combine baking soda and the essential oil.
- Put the mixture in the refrigerator in an open container to absorb any smells.

Steps to clean using citrus fridge deodorizer;

- Clean up spills right away to make cleaning easier and avoid bacterial contamination.

Cleaning the Microwave

In as much as microwaves can clean itself. It is also essential for you to clean it to have a better-cleaned microwave.

Quick-And-Easy Microwave Cleaner

To form Quick-And-Easy Microwave Cleaner, do the following;

- 2 part of white distilled vinegar
- 2 part of a water

Then to clean your microwave using the Quick-And-Easy Microwave cleaner, do the following;

- Mix the vinegar and water in a microwave-safe bowl.
- Microwave on high for a few minutes.

We expect that the mixture will aid the softening of any food plaster in the microwave.

- Remove carefully the bowl (both the bowl and the liquid will be boiling)
- Make use of soft cloth and an all-purpose spray of your choice to clean out the microwave.

- To clean the microwave outside, use any all-purpose sprays of your choice.

- In a situation where the location of your microwave is above the stove, make sure you periodically take off any vents or filters and clean them thoroughly.

To clean a burn on top of your stovetop;

- Pour hot water on it.

- Allow the hot water to sit for some minutes.

- Then finally clean the top of the stove with a towel

Glass Stove Cleaner

Another way you can clean your stove or oven is by using a Glass Stove Cleaner, which is formed by combining the following;

- 2 part of baking soda
- 2 part of fine salt
- 2 part of a water

Combine all these ingredients to create a paste. Apply the paste on the top of the glass stove and let it sit. Finally, scrub the dirt out with a clean cloth.

Hot Water Stove Cleaner

Another way you can clean your stove or oven is by using a Hot Water Stove Cleaner;

I know this will sound ridiculous to you, but know that nothing cleans your dirt from the top of a stove better than hot water.

To achieve this, follow the following steps;

- Pour hot water on the stovetop
- Let it soften the food.
- Wipe the top of the stove using a soft cloth,

You can do this in combination with any all-purpose sprays of your choice to kill any remaining bacteria.

Note: if the water you are using is hot enough, you can even skip the process of using an all-purpose spray.

Oven Cleaner

To form your oven cleaner,

- Use warm or hot water
- Baking soda
- Orange essential oil

Through this step, you can clean your oven by

- We are adding warm/hot water to baking soda to get a loose paste.
- Put a few drops of essential oil for scent.
- Put the combination of dirty areas of the oven.
- Allow the paste to sit for 15–30 minutes.
- With hot water + scrub brush, thoroughly clean the oven.

Note that there is some oven cleaner out there in the toxic market; instead of using those cleaner, you can make use of 100% Natural Multi-purpose Cleaner, or you use hot water mixed with a baking soda paste in your oven. Allow to sit for some minute and scrub gently to remove a stain.

Now that you discover the secrets of making a kitchen green cleaner yourself. It is time to take a step and make one for yourself not only for the safety of your health but for the safety of your family. The reason you need to take this seriously is because of the likeliness of the manufactured cleaning agent sold in the market to cause cancer because of the presence of the carcinogenic ingredient that is used during its manufacturing process.

Therefore to keep yourself safe, your family, friends, and everyone around you safe, you have to take the best bold step and make this organic cleaning product yourself and start living a healthy life while your kitchen is kept clean.

To get access to my A-Z formula for making organic cleaner for your city room and offices, send "Need" to godwinchigozie679@gmail.com to get the book.